Acid Reflux Solution

By

Dermot Farrell

www.healbodymindandspirit.com

MEDICAL DISCLAIMER

The information in this book is not intended to replace professional medical supervision. Acid reflux is a potentially serious health condition and should be regarded with respect. The information in this book is highly effective and it will definitely reduce the acid reflux of nearly every person, who earnestly uses the techniques outlined within. In some cases a cure may take place; however, there is no guarantee that acid reflux will be completely cured. Prior to reducing or stopping acid reflux medications do consult with a qualified physician.

Contents

Introduction

Are you tired of having heartburn yet again?

Have you tried out every "cure" under the Sun to find yourself still having problems with acid reflux?

Have you suffered with an "iffy" stomach, most of your adult life and with no apparent possibility for relief!

Well you don't have to be!

Acid reflux is either brushed off as a minor irritation (when in fact it can be a major irritation if you get it regularly), or it's labelled as a disease (GERD – Gastroesophageal Reflux Disease), when in reality acid reflux is a symptom caused by an unbalanced body!

In this guidebook you will be given an overview as to how and what acid reflux is, followed by a variety of strategies which can both reduce symptoms and in some cases, over a period of time, a complete cure can take place.

You shall read about how to eat the right way, so as to reduce stomach acid problems; breathing exercises to reduce the onset of acid reflux; helpful natural herbs and healthy supplements which will help and physical exercises, including hatha yoga and oriental energetic exercises.

Take a quick look through this book and you can find some helpful strategies, which will help both to reduce the frequency and intensity of acid reflux events and if you get a little deeper into it, by observing yourself and making the appropriate long term changes that a cure will be possibly for many, or at least a great reduction in symptomology!

Chapter One – Acid Reflux – What is It? – What to do About It?

Acid reflux is one of those annoying modern health conditions which don't appear to have a common cause, yet it upsets millions of people year on year.

So let's take a closer look:

Acid Reflux/heartburn

If you Google acid reflux you will get the same definition for acid reflux which is:

Acid reflux is a burning sensation which is felt internally in the lower chest area. The acid reflux is simply the stomach acid refluxing up the walls of the stomach into the oesophagus, while the heart burn is the name attached to the symptoms of burning sensation which goes along with the acid reflux.

GERD

GERD (Gastroesophageal **reflux** disease) is simply a label attached to anyone who regularly undergoes a bout of acid reflux more than twice a week!

The Causes of Acid Reflux/Heart Burn/GERD

Once again if you Google the causes of acid reflux you will probably come up with an extensive list which runs like this:

- Smoking

- Obesity

- Low fibre intake

- High intake of salt

- Lack of physical exercise

- High Alcohol or caffeine intake

- Some over the counter medications

The problem with this listing approach is that it all about labels but there are no explanations as to why a person should have higher than normal acid levels in their stomachs. It is true the people who are obese, heavy smokers etc. will be more prone to developing acid reflux, because these bad habits are putting they're bodies out of synch, thus resulting in many health imbalances of which acid reflux is just one of them.

Acid Reflux from a Complementary Health Perspective

Most gastrointestinal doctors will simply talk at length about genetics and bad lifestyle choices, resulting in too much stomach acid. But there is opposite and indeed contrarian point of view which I would like you to consider and it's this:

A person who suffers with acid reflux symptoms is a person who has lower than average acid levels in the stomach!

Because of imbalances which are largely lifestyle related, but can also be caused by genetics, some people are more inclined towards developing acid reflux symptoms, but really what's actually happening is that they are too low on stomach acid. Because of imbalances the stomach is not making enough stomach acid!

But how can someone having too low stomach acid levels result in acid reflux?

The answer to this is simple, because the stomach lacks acid it attempts to produce more acid, but the increase in acid levels are not balanced, rather the acid levels fluctuate and are sporadic resulting in too little aid to digest the food properly and then large dollops of stomach acid are released and they bypass the stomach altogether and go straight to the oesophagus. The oesophagus is not designed to deal with stomach acid, so once the stomach acid finds its way there the results in burning and with that comes burning pain!

The Difference between the Allopathic and Complementary Assessment of Acid Reflux

So simply put the allopathic viewpoint is that acid reflux results from too much stomach acid, but they only like to list of possible lifestyle causes, but not actual biological causes, whereas complementary medicine suggests that your acid reflux problems are caused by too little hydrochloric acid in the stomach, which results in the body producing intermittent supplies of the acid, which in turn burns the oesophagus.

I like a lot of things about western (allopathic) medicine, because often the drugs can be very helpful, but also sometimes allopathic approach can be a silly approach and we see this clearly with acid reflux.

If you go down to your local GP and complain about acid reflux, they will give you some antacid tabs. If the condition continues, they shall write a prescription for more antacids and possibly some tests, and even after the tests results come back and you end up meeting with a gastrointestinal specialist you will still end up getting some more powerful antacids!

You have an acid problem with your stomach because of an unbalanced lifestyle and yes antacids can help, but not in the long-term, in the long-term you have to make lifestyle changes and rebalance the subtle energies in your body. By all means use the allopathic approach as a stop gap mechanism, by way of using antacids to reduce the inflammation, but use complementary medicine to cure your acid reflux!

There are a variety of approaches which you can take to alleviate acid reflux. The good news is that there are lots of options available to you and as chronic conditions go acidic reflux is more treatable than most. However on the downside acid reflux can take time to cure, because acid reflux can arise whenever there is a big imbalance somewhere in the gastrointestinal tract. Just take a look at this diagram of the gastrointestinal tract and you can see how it begins with the mouth, becomes the oesophagus, then the stomach, then large and finally small intestines and then rectum. The purpose of these extensive structures is to break down food so that the body can thrive on the energy which it imbibes from the food it has eaten. But the problem is that imbalances can occur anywhere, dude of the sheer complexity of the gastrointestinal tract!

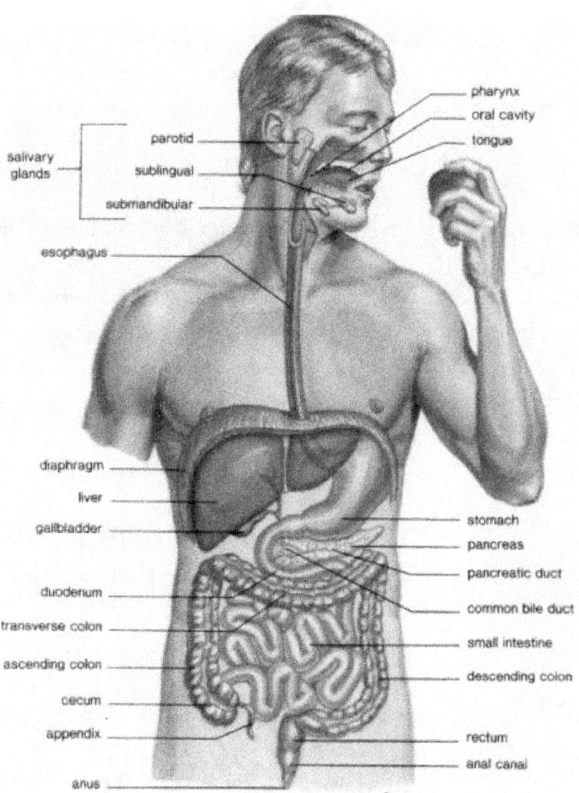

For example, say you eat too much food and your intestines are backed up with undigested food, this could result in a slow evacuation of food from the stomach which in turn could help to promote irregular stomach acid activity. However, another variation on this theme could a person who eats little, but the foods they eat are antagonistic to the gastrointestinal system. For example, a person might like really spicy food, but this food ends up burning the lining of the stomach and the intestines and once again over time an imbalance occurs and irregular acid levels arise followed by acid reflux!

So there's no one way to get acid reflux. If you want to cure acid reflux permanently, then it's very important that you observe yourself and see under what conditions you suffer from acid reflux and this should give you some clue as to what imbalance you are facing. For example, a lot of heavy drinkers skip eating solid meals and get by on a diet almost solely consisting of alcohol, so obviously such outlandish behaviour as living on alcohol or eating very spicy chillies every day of the week, are extremely foolish as it will result in inflammation of the stomach wall and possible intestines and should be avoided, what other triggers are present?

For a lot of people the most major trigger will be food type. Often if I go and eat at a 4 or 5 star hotel I will get some acid reflux and I think the reason is because been middle aged the levels of enzymes in my gastrointestinal tract are a little on the low side, which is to be expected as enzyme levels start to drop off with age, for anyone over the age of 30. This combination of lower enzyme levels combined with food which taste great but which are high in fats and strong additives, designed to make the food taste healthy, end up putting a strain on the GI system. For a start these foods are extremely high in calories, so a serving which would normally be a 1000 calorie Meal turns into a 2500 calories meal, thanks to the density of the fats and carbs in these foods and then add in the additives and lower enzyme levels in there and acid reflux here I come!

So what do I do to cure or prevent acid reflux?

Well first of all I avoid eating very rich hotel type food most of the time, simply eating homemade foods works a treat for me. Secondly, if I eat this rich food or spicy food, I will try and get my hands on some natural yoghurt.

Natural Yoghurt Treatment

Natural yoghurt is a base, so this helps with acidity but also it's high on friendly probiotics, which are healthy and helpful bacteria. Natural yoghurt will almost instantly treat the symptoms of acid reflux, and while it won't cure acid reflux, it's a great and natural way of balancing your stomach acids quickly. Also a distinct advantage of natural yoghurt is that if you eat say 500grams (around a pint) of natural yoghurt, it will take a few minutes to eat this yoghurt and each time you take a spoonful your adding cooling refreshing yoghurt into your oesophagus, which is great. Whereas if you take an antacid pill or an antacid solution, it gives relief but it's all over in a few seconds. So before you reach for your antacids, try out a tub of natural ypughuirt first and see how you get on!

Inflammationary Problems

Probably one of the biggest causes of acid reflux is intestinal inflammation and inflammation of the stomach lining. There are many reasons why this happens but often these imbalances come about as a consequence of eating foods which are highly toxic and the body tries to protect itself by responding to the toxicity via a chain reaction, which results in inflammation. Initially the inflammation protects against the toxicity, but over time the inflammation causes its own problems, because that organ (gastointesteintla tract in this case) can no longer function effectively!

In particular **LEAKY GUT SYNDROME** will usually kick in. **LEAKY GUT SYNDROME (LKS)** is a complex health condition, whereby the discrete separation between healthy nutrients and toxins within the intestinal lining become mixed with the result that the health of the entire body becomes undermined!

If we go back and look at the diagram of the GI system, we see the stomach, small intestines and large intestines taking centre stage. Well the stomach helps to break down the food, so that it becomes an easy digestible liquid called "chyme" and the large intestines are really only for evacuation of waste. The most important work takes place in the small intestines. Now from a physical point of view, when we feel hungry we feel that our stomachs are empty and we feel good when our stomachs are full. Because of this we tend to think that our stomachs are digesting the food, but this is not actually true, rather the stomach is for predigestion only. Rather it's the small intestines which absorb the nutrients. The problem, however from an LKS point of view, is that it's the small intestines where food is absorbed and also it's the small intestines where toxins get pulled out and processed or in some cases simply evacuated down through the large intestines. Everything works fine as long as there is a discrete separation of nutrients versus toxins, but in LKS this gets mixed up, the body starts taking in toxins in an unabsorbed state and the body react via inflammation, in an effort to cordon off the damage!

Energetic Imbalances

My background is in Traditional Chinese Medicine (TCM) and Chinese medicine isn't just about putting needles into body parts, it's mainly about energetic imbalances and using various techniques to get that balance back.

The idea in TCM is that energy moves on channels (meridians) and that there are points on these channels which can either raise lower energy levels, reduce energy levels which is excessive or stimulate stagnant energy into moving in a balanced way. So whatever health problem we have, it always goes back to rebalancing.

In the case of gastrointestinal problems, the stomach, spleen and kidney energies will be the main meridians which will be out of balance. So another approach, which we can try to help treat our acid reflux is to look at the energetic balance of our body's and by doing so we can also go a long way towards bringing about health and balance!

To summarise, there are lots of approaches which we can take, the important thing been to realise the difference between treating acid reflux and curing it. From the point of view of treating it we can do a few things right and we will improve the symptoms. But to cure our acid reflux then we has to restore the balance within our bodies.

If you make a concerted effort to restore the balance within your body, you can definitely cure acid reflux, even GERT, if you're determined but its takes time (as in months in severe cases) but it can be done. You will always be prone to acid reflux, once you have had it repeatedly, but you will be able to cure it and prevent further attacks, so long as you're willing to make life changes and follow the advice in the following chapters regarding rebalancing your gastrointestinal health!

Chapter Three – General Advice Regarding Eating to Prevent and Treat Stomach Acid Reflux

In this chapter some information from my book Gut health is presented because it's just as relevant in this book as it is in the Gut Health book. Simply put the number one way to avoid developing stomach acidity is to eat right in the first place. There is a tendency amongst most people to eat according to their palate and not their stomach. Have you ever noticed yourself eating a sumptuous meal only to find your stomach complaining instantly, well this is an obvious case of our taste buds liking the food but our gut disliking it!

By way of example, I love ice cream and I have a tendency when I eat ice cream (which is probably once every month or two or three) to eat too much. When I begin to eat the ice cream I feel a nice soothing sensation in my stomach, but once I get onto my second bowl, I start to feel a distension in my stomach and a tendency towards weakness. Now I won't get acid reflux from eating ice cream, but definitely when eating in excess, it results in an undermining of my stomach which could result in other imbalances in my stomach, possibly the next day or two after eating excess ice creams. It just goes to show you that it's not as simple as "oh I ate a chilly and now I have acid reflux". Ok it is this simple in some cases, if for example, you look up chilly challenge on You Tube, you shall see a vast array of foolish people who are challenging themselves to eat really hot chillies and I think that acid reflux is probably the least of their problems, as they gyrate around their kitchens with their eyes bulging from their sockets and they are coughing and gasping for dear life! So clearly a case of excess!

But in the case of acid reflux, often we undermine our stomachs over time, which makes them more prone to producing intermittent levels of stomach acid, which is also added to an inflamed stomach lining and intestinal lining and often

18

a bloated gaseous environment, which all leads towards acid reflux. So take a look at this chapter and try to amend any bad habits which you are having regarding general eaten habits, get the basics right first and then add in the beiger changes later as needs be!

Simple Food Advice

Probably the single biggest factor which causes an unbalanced gut is diet. I think we all know about this but it can be difficult to change our diet. However, at least we have to try and be sensible. Just take a trip down to your local supermarket/minimarket and have a look around at most of the foodstuffs present therein. If you try to take an objective look at what you see, rather than simply reacting out of habit, you will notice that around 80% of the food available is either junk (as in biscuits, cakes, ice creams, sodas and so forth), or it might as well be junk as in its highly processed foods. For example most cereals and breads are highly processed as too are dairy products. Fish is usually bookish, so long as it's not salmon (as farmed salmon is often high in toxins) or canned fish.

Meat on the other hand is a veritable war zone of injected hormones and chemicals, so most of this is also junk. So what you are left with is the vegetables and fruits, most of which has been over fertilised and often picked and frozen, shipped half way around the world and stored in freezer for an indeterminate period of time! The average apple available in most American super markets, for example, will be up to six months old!

Fresh orange juice is often made from a pulp, which has a whole bunch of additives mixed in there, and it too has usually been in the deep freeze for a mini-ice age!

And just because it tastes good and appears authentic doesn't mean anything. By and large most foods, even the apparently fresh ones have been processed weeks or even months before we have gotten our hands on them. And even good old organic cannot be trusted. Most organic food is not as organic as you might think. Basically unless you bought it direct from the farm, there is no way to know whether it is really fresh (versus deep frozen for a period of time) or that it really is organic!

I'm not saying this to depress you, after all I also buy food from my local supermarket, and unless you live in a region surrounded by organic farmers, where you can buy produce direct from them or you have big cash reserves, whereby you can buy the highest quality food from a top quality health food store, then you just have to get on with eating a bunch of denatured food!

However, while it is virtually impossible these days to have access to the best quality food, at least we can try and steer things into the right direction. For example, if you have a farmers market near you, try and buy fruits and vegetables there. There is a good chance that the food is not organic but there is a good chance that it's actually fairly fresh. Try and buy organic fruit and vegetables from trusted sources, if you can find them. Also wash both fruit and vegetables thoroughly, so as to get some of the chemicals of off them prior to eating them and finally have a look at your eating habits and try to reduce dependence on processed foods where possible.

While it would be ideal to live on an organic farm and eat everything fresh from Mother Nature, this is probably not going to be the reality for most of us. However, I do believe that even if the food isn't organic and it's probably deep frozen etc., that at least where most of our food intake is home prepared instead of out of a bag or a box, that chances are that it's reasonably healthy. Try where possible to eat as much fruit and vegetables as you can and try to eat raw where possible. As raw food, especially raw vegetables and fruits are high in enzymes (at least some of the time depending upon deep freezing etc.). So at least when we prepare our own food, we are not adding in a bunch of preservatives and additives.

The thing to remember with the modern food industry is that it's all about making money and the way to do this is to make everything appear fresh even if it's not. Think about it this way, if you go into your local store and you buy a fruit or a vegetable that's out of season, then how can it be available unless it has been deep frozen? If you buy a fruit or vegetable, which isn't readily available in your country, then it has been picked from some other country and usually shipped over, in which case it's many weeks or months old!

So one simple way to try and maintain a healthy diet, is to try to eat food according to season, because chances are that if it's in season, then there is a good chance that its actually fresh!

21

Another thing with the food industry is of course preservatives and additives, so that all those nice tasty foods present in jars, tins, packets and bags are all nice and fresh, many months after they are purchased. So keeping them fresh artificially is good for business, but it's bad for the consumer as we take this crap into our body's, over time toxins build up which make it difficult for our gut to cope with them!

So following on from the old adage that prevention is the best cure, try where possible to eat organic, ideally from the farm and even if this is not possible, try your best to tip the balance over towards eating foods, which are home prepared rather than highly processed, regardless how good they taste.

Finally if we take a look at sources of macronutrients, namely proteins, carbohydrates and fats, we have to take a look at how we are getting these micronutrients. For example in many western countries, huge amounts of bread and dairy products have been the mainstay of diets for centuries. However, most bread today, for example, isn't what it used to be rather it's usually full of cheap starches, even if it appears to be multi-grain; often the multi-grain is more or less a cosmetic after thought. Just make some brown bread at home and compare it to multi-grain, from your local shop, and see how you feel after five or six slices of each and you will notice some discomfort and bloating with the supermarket multi-grain versus homemade. I know that everyone cannot bake their own bread and that supermarket multi-grain, is far better than supermarket white bread, but it's still not great.

22

Dairy is also questionable, since it's heavily processed versus raw milk and dairy products which have been made on the farm. So I know it can be difficult or even impossible to change these things, but at least we should reduce our dependency upon them. For example, growing up in Ireland, vast quantities of white bread, cheese, processed milk and endless cereals was the name of the game and this is a recipe for gut problems. Because processed bread is starchy, milk and dairy products are full of lactose (unless you are using raw milk which can be hard to get your hands on). So even if you cannot stop taking these foodstuffs, at least reduce your dependency on them.

When I was growing up about 75% of all the food, which I was eating, could be classified under these groups and this sort of highly processed food, combined with a lack of fruit and vegetables in the diet will result in gut problems!

Also in Asian countries rice is very popular which is fine? But rice up to about 60 years ago was heavy organic rice, which was yellow in colour and had a thick outer husk, which is highly nutritious. But modern processed rice has been denatured, in the same way that processed white sugar has been denatured. They have thrown out the outer husk and what you left with as a highly polished, tasty and fairly un-nutritious white grain. It looks pretty but it's not that healthy. So where possible go for organic rice, but most organic rice isn't even really organic. But at least you can reduce your dependency on rice. These days I live in India and a lot of pole in South India eat pounds of rice per day, which is too much. Many of them have distended stomachs, because just like beer drinkers in the west develop stomach distension, so too do many Asian people develop stomach distension.

I'm not suggesting that you give up your favourite foods, but just realise that different cultures have developed a dependence upon certain kinds of food, which has come about historically. But these foods are not the same food which we are using today, so for a start bread, dairy, rice and other cereals where far healthier pre-world war II. Secondly, we tend to eat more foods these days and thirdly we are less active than we sued to be. So because grandpa used to eat a truck load of bread and dairy 60 years ago, when the food was all organic and he worked doing physical labour on the farm for 10 hours a day, whereby his body was like a furnace and burnt off all of the carbohydrates and calories, so of course he was healthy. But now we are eating the same food while leaving a sedentary lifestyle, eating denatured food and lots of it!

Consequently we have to change some of our historical eating patterns, because for a start we don't need such a volume of food. Back in the old days a farmer or manual labourer could easily eat a 1000 grams of carbohydrates a day and burn it off, because they needed 5000 plus calories a day, because of psychical work. If you are a sedentary office worker, then chances are that you will only need somewhere between 2000 to 3000 calories of total food per day, depending upon gender and physical side and general activity levels. So we have to take a look at our food habits and make some changes.

Also because so much of these stable food items are now just junk, probably the easiest way to relieve our digestive systems is to get a little built creative and try to eat a variety of foods, so as to give our gut a chance. If we're eating a pound of bread a day or two pounds of rice a day or a pound of cereals per day or a pound of cheese and other dairy products a day, it's just a bit much for our digestive system to deal with. The simplest way to give your digestive system a break is to give it a variety of foods, ideally in a balanced way which includes vegetables and fruits. Chances are that when we eat a variety of foods, even if these foods are not organic, that we get a better variety of macro and micronutrients and also it puts less pressure on out guts, as eating vast quantities of the one food, requires a lot of the same sort of enzymes to break it down. So when we eat vast quantities of one kind of food, even if organic, it ends up in a backlog of undigested food in our gut and sometimes even the development of an allergy to that kind of food!

General Good Eating Habits

Before taking a look at supplements for people who are having gut problems, we should first of all remind ourselves to check our eating habits, as it's not just the food you eat but also how you eat which is really important. According to hatha yogis we should chew our food 44 times before swallowing!

I know if we all did this, we would be very slim (because we would not be eating much food) and we would have really big lower faces (thanks to our huge masseter muscles), but on a more practical note, we should at least make a point of chewing our food. I remember when I was young, my brother Tony mastered the art of eating and swallowing a full sized Cities digestive biscuit (it's about 2.5 inches in diameter) in one go and while it was entertaining to watch, this is obviously not a good way to eat our food. Yet most of us do something similar most of the time. In our busy society our tendency is to eat our food in gulp like fashion, as if we haven't seen food for several days and had to satisfy our hanger. Another aspect of modern food eating habits is to sit over our food face down and rat like pigs in a through, we gulp our food down as if are in a race to see who finishes first!

Chew Your Food Thoroughly: Well these are all really bad food eating habits. While it may not be practical or even enjoyable to chew our food for 44 times, we should at least be cognizant that we are eating our food and chew it according to texture. Something like oats or rice pudding can be swallowed, without any really chewing as they are already semi-solid in nature, but foods like meat, fish, bread, biscuits etc., should be chewed and broken down into a semi solid, prior to leaving our mouth. Looking at Mother Nature, this is what our salivary glands are for. The idea is to have the saliva break the food down in our mouth so that it is semi-solid, then the stomach acid makes it more liquid, so it become a soup like substance, called chime and finally this liquid substance filters through the intestines delivering nutrients as it goes.

So the first step to good gut health is good digestion, and this means chewing our food. Gobbling down great big chunks of red meat, for instance, is really putting stress on our gut. If we take a look at a typical western styled lunch of baguette filled with chicken, for example, when we gulp this down bits of chicken and bread are sitting in our stomachs and since the stomach empties its content within about 20 minutes, the chunks of bread and chicken are still only semi-solid. No wonder the intestine gets back logged and this can be particular severe on foods such as red meat, which are notorious for festering inside the intestines and take at least 24 hours to digest and sometimes more. This is also why it is good to take a variety of meats, over the course of a week, as red meat in particular is difficult to digest. Also some vegetarian foods are famously difficult to digest with noodles been slow to digest, for example.

Anyhow the first step to gut health is to watch your diet and the second is to chew your food, so as to give your gut a chance to properly digest it.

Eating and Activity: Another aspect of eating food is activity. These days I see lots of people eating while walking, for instance, which makes no sense at all as it makes digestion difficult. Another thing is eating while sitting at our desk feeling stressed. For a start we are probably bent over our desk which makes digestion difficult and worrying or stressing, while eating is a real no!

From a Traditional Chinese medical (TCM) point of view, we should eat in a relaxed and conscious manner, we should be aware that we are eating and enjoy and feel the nurturing effects, as this boosts both yang (active) and yang (nurturing) energy. While this sounds esoteric, it is in fact a very common sense approach to eating, as conscious awareness helps us to relax, which in turn will relax our digestive system; also we will eat more slowly thus allowing our digestive enzymes and stomach acid to do their work and we will feel more contented, which in turn will make us less likely to eat too much. Often times when we rush through our food, we don't even notice that we are eating and end up eating more. Have you ever ate an ice cream or a chocolate bar, only to find out that the last bite was the tastiest and you wish you had more? Chances are you gobbled down the treat so quickly, that you only consciously noticed that you were eating chocolate or ice cream, when you imbibed your last mouth full!

Water Intake at Mealtime: Other good food device is to watch our water intake prior to and post food intake. Our stomach is an acid bath and if we drink water either just before or just after food, we end up diluting the acid, which in turn limits the digestibility of the food. You can of course take milk or other beverages, as they will either be acids or bases, but don't take water with your meal as its ph. neutral so it will put the stomach of!

Another good piece of eating advice is to eat less rather than more. In Japan, for example, the people of the Islands of Okinawa are famous for their longevity. There are several factors, which help them live such a long life, but one of the major factors recognised is that they eat until they are still slightly hungry. The brain takes 15 minutes to catch up with the stomach, so if you stop eating when you are full, about 15 minutes later you will feel really bloated! So there is some real wisdom in the Okinawans approach to eating!

Who hasn't eaten too much food at Christmas, thanksgiving or at a birthday party or in a restaurant while on holidays, but let's be honest is it good for health?

Certainly not, as lying on our bed feeling like a beached whale, for a few hours, is not a pleasant way to spend our afternoon or evening and think about the damage which is been done to our gut. The food is simply backing up and been undigested thus making the entire digestive system run badly. You can do it now and again and get away with it, but if you repeatedly abuse your gut, it will bite back with a variety of gut health issues!

Avoid Spicy Food: Another good
piece of advice is to avoid very spicy foods. I know some people love eating
spicy food, but spicy food especially if mixed with hard liquor is a recipe for
disaster, as it will mess up your stomach! Also another consideration is to balance
spicy with non-spicy. In India, for example, spicy food is popular, but so is eating
rice mixed with curd (natural yoghurt) at the end of the meal. The thing about
natural yoghurt is that it is a base and it neutralises the acidic effects of spice. So
yoghurt or milk is good foods to help wash down a spicy meal, and whatever you
do don't drink water when eating spicy food. You Tube is full of entries of
people swallowing hot chillies and then trying to recover by drinking water, well
water actually reignites the spice and makes things worse! Next time you eat
something too spicy at the restaurant, order a glass or milk or natural yoghurt
and forget about the water as it will do more harm than good!

Eat Frequently: Eating
frequently is another good protocol. Although most of us like to binge these
days, our bodies actually like to eat little but often. Although this can vary from
person to person, as some people do better on fewer meals, for the majority of
people eating little but often makes the digestive system run well, it helps to
maintain metabolic levels and keep nutrients running around the body.

Don't eat late at night. Back in Ireland it's a popular past time for many people go to the pub and drink alcohol, followed by the inevitable take away as beer encourages appetite. But this is a disastrous decision, as one pint of beer contains around 200 calories, so say 4 pints of beer equals 800 calories, all of which are carbohydrates. Then add in another 1500 calories, in the form of a burger, French fries and a bottle of coke and you are now looking at a days' worth of calories followed by sleep!

This is a crazy idea as the liver goes asleep at around 10pm in the evening. Large intakes of calories, just before sleep, will bloat you while you sleep and leave you hungry when you wake up, for the food hasn't been processed. Then when you wake up, you eat more which encourages weight gain and a backlog of food in the intestines!

The same also goes for non-drinkers. Say you work night shift, well don't come home at 5am and eat a big meal and then sleep, rather eat something small and have a really big meal when you wake up, it will work out far better for your body. The human body is designed to process food during daylight hours, so try as best you can to keep most of you're eating between 6am and 6pm where possible, at a push you can still eat till around 9pm at night, but definitely eating later than that is a serious no for most people's digestive systems!

Hydrate: Finally back to water again, do drink enough water, as in at least 1 litter (2 pints) a day, and this could be as high as 10 litters (20 pints) depending upon climate. While some people suggest that water is not important, actually it is.

Have you ever felt thirsty after a meal? Well the reason why is because digestion uses water, if you want to digest your food you have to drink water. The best policy is to sip water throughout the day. Also carbohydrates suck in water. Every gram of carbohydrates brings along 4 grams of water along with it, so if you are eating a lot, you have to take in a lot of water, otherwise the body will become dehydrated!

There are a wide variety of herbs and supplements which you can take to help reduce your acid reflux symptoms and in some cases long-term exposure may well help to cure acid reflux. For example, ginger helps the stomach to evacuate food faster, which in turn aids digestion and L-Glutamine is an amino acid which helps to repair damage to the stomach and intestinal lining, which again over time might help to cure acid reflux.

The material which follows is quite varied in character and it covers herbs and supplements for stomach and intestinal health and not just acid reflux. Experiment and see which ones work well for you!

Ginger

Ginger is a popular food supplement, but also it is a wondrous herb which has many great traits one of which is on digestion. In a clinical study on the effectiveness of ginger on speeding up the breakdown of food in the stomach, they took 24 participants and gave them 1.2grams of ginger one hour prior to eating a meal and then observed how long it took for the food to transit from the stomach into the intestines. Normally it will take approximately 20 minutes for the food to transit, however the average figure which came back in this group was a transit time of only 13 minutes. 1 This indicates that the ginger helped the food predigest approximately 50% faster than normal. What this suggests is that ginger will help food to predigest, which will in turn make for better chyme and thus an easier time on the intestines when it comes to absorbing the food.

Furthermore ginger also helps relieve symptoms of nausea. In another clinical trial on 32 pregnant ladies, who were suffering with morning sickness, they were given 1 gram of ginger per day and by the end of the study 28 out of the 32 women noticed a significant reduction in morning sickness symptoms![2]

So ginger not only helps to breakdown the food but also it helps to settle the stomach, in cases of people who are prone to stomach upset!

There are lots of ways to take ginger. After all you can add ginger into your cooking, but one very effective and tasty way to take ginger is as a tea.

Ginger Tea

1. Take 250ml of water (8 ounces) and add in several slices of ginger, taken directly from ginger root. Simply take some ginger root (about 3 grams per cup) and peel of the outer layer of skin from one part of it and then cut of several slices. Take these slices and either crush slightly or blend in a mix for a few seconds before adding into the water. Another approach is to pound them slightly in a pewter, as once the ginger is crushed a little, its helpful compounds will be released.

2. Boil the water and leave to simmer for a good 10 to 15 minutes, in order to get the essence of ginger out. When we think about boiling vegetables versus steaming, steaming is always recommended because boiling takes out the nutrients from the vegetables and puts it into the water, whereas steaming does not do this. However, in this case we want the nutrients within the ginger to come out into the water as we are going to drink it!

3. You will know the tea is ready when a distinct ginger aroma is smelt.

4. Put a tablespoon of honey into a cup

5. Take one small lemon or half a medium sized lemon and squeeze into the same cup

6. Strain the now boiled ginger water into the cup which has honey and lemon present. If you have done a good job, the tea should be strong enough to sting your throat a little but, this means that you really have got the essence of ginger with all of its amazing benefits!

7. Other options include adding in cinnamon and cardamom, which not only add taste but also they add enormous national benefits as well.

For a video on how to make ginger tea click here:

<u>How to Make Ginger tea Video</u>

For more information on the powerful effects of ginger and other great herbs, check out my book

"<u>Medicinal herbs</u>"

Peppermint

Peppermint has a calming effect on an upset stomach. It relaxes the muscles of the stomach and helps increase the flow of bile. In particular peppermint has a good effect on symptoms of nausea. In a study on the effects of peppermint on post-operative nausea found that peppermint made a significant improvement in nauseas symptoms in patients who took it.3

Furthermore, peppermint helps relieve irritable bowel syndrome (IBS), due to its ability to relax the intestinal walls. Peppermints ability to relax gastrointestinal muscles, means that it is a good way to treat stomach aches, nausea and constipation.

Regarding dosing peppermint is usually taken as a tea and peppermint tea is commonly found in many health food stores and even supermarkets. Of course you can always make your own peppermint tea as follows;

Peppermint Tea

1. Boil water

2. Add in some peppermint leaves

3. Boil for 10 minutes

4. Strain and serve

Wheatgrass is awesome yet underrated herb which can really help gut health. Wheatgrass is simply the grass which becomes wheat, being chopped when the grass is only 6 inches in height. Anyway this grass possesses many amazing benefits which include the following benefits:

- Balances the body's Ph. Levels
- Deoxygenates our bodies
- Protects against cancer
- Boosts red blood cell count
- Cleanses the blood
- Liver detoxification
- Improves digestion
- Extremely high in nutrients including vitamins A, B6, C, K and E, manganese, selenium, copper and zinc
- Very high in dietary fibre
- Thyroid stimulation
- Promotes weight loss
- Strengthens bones
- Regulates blood sugar levels
- Improves blood lipid levels
- Increases athletic performance

Wheatgrass is so potent that it's worth taking as a great health booster and everyone should really take it for a couple of reasons. First of all our diet is very acidic these days, as foods such as cereals, milk and dairy products are all acidic. Most foods which are bases are vegetables, so unless you are eating a truck load of vegetables, your body is probably going to be too acidic. Our bodies are meant to operate slightly into the base range of around 7.35-7.45. The Ph. Scale runs from 0 to 6 which is most acidic to least acidic, with coke and coffee being around 4, on this scale and then we have water which is Ph. Neutral, which is 7 and then we go from 8, which is least base, to 14 which is most base. So our bodies are meant to be slightly base. Our bloodstream has to maintain this narrow range of 7.35 to 7.45, and in order to maintain this level our body will even bleach minerals out of our bones, in an effort to maintain this narrow range in our bloodstream!

Now aside from immanent death, which would happen if our bloodstreams Ph. levels ran outside of this narrow range, even when our body manages to artificially maintain this blood level balance, the body in general is too acidic and in extreme cases this can result in acidosis, where a variety of complaints can arise which includes:

- Fatigue
- Drowsiness
- Shortness of breath
- Headaches
- Confusion
- Tremors

If you have some of these symptoms, then chances are that you either have acidosis or are on the way there. Few people develop full-blown acidosis, but lots of people suffer from borderline acidosis whereby they have aches and pains, feel fatigued and drained and generally their bodies are not working well.

So what has this got to do with gut issues?

Well while gut Ph. level has to be acidic, the body in general should be base, in order to function efficiently. For example, an acidic environment promotes fungal growth, bacterial growth and viral growth, within the body. When we get our Ph. Levels back into the normal range, this bodily environment isn't suitable for funguses, bacteria or viruses. So getting rid of these pathogenic invaders helps amongst other things a healthy gut. The great thing with wheatgrass is that it helps to get the Ph.levels back inline without resorting to eating large quantities of vegetables each day..

Also wheatgrass is high in fructans which promote lactobacilli (healthy gut bacteria – which aid digestion and help to kill of nasty funguses such as Candida, for example) and they also help promote reabsorption of calcium, which promotes bones health, lowers triglyceride levels, which aids heart health and helps to reduce blood glucose levels.

Another great benefit of wheatgrass is its high micronutrient level, which promotes once again digestive health and finally wheatgrass is very high in soluble fibre, to the degree that ingesting wheatgrass can promote bowel movements, especially in people who are having gut health issues.

Wheatgrass is a great herb and will boost your health in general, but certainly it has a great benefit on gut health. Importantly when you initially take wheatgrass,

39

usually it will have as strong effect on bowel movements. So when you start taking wheatgrass at first, don't be surprised if you end up suddenly having to go to the toilet. Fortunately this will right itself within a few days or weeks. The good news however, is that its' your gut righting itself and the reason why there are so many bowel movements is because the wheatgrass is moving stubborn blockages within the intestines. So getting as this 'crap' (literarily) gets thrown out of our bodies, which is really good for health and most people, who have gut health issues, nearly always there will be a backlog, so moving this backlog is the first step towards good gut health. Also for people who are suffering with diarrhoea, wheatgrass will help to balance the healthy gut bacteria which will have the reverse effect of normalising bowel movements!

Regarding how to take wheatgrass, ideally you should grow your own, but this tends to be a big hassle, so while the organic, made at home in your garden wheatgrass is the best, even still the powder form which you get in your local health store, is still pretty good and well worth your while to take it.

To take wheatgrass in powder form, just take two tablespoons (30 grams) of it and add in around 250 ml (8 ounces) of water, stir with a spoon and drink. If you have been having lots of stomach health issues, then take this 3 times a day initially, but when things settle down, take just once a day, as this is enough to greatly promote gut health and health in general!

Apple Cider Vinegar (ACV) goes hand in hand with wheatgrass in that it is a powerful general health elixir and also it is very good for gut health. The benefits of ACV includes the following:

- Balances the bodies Ph. Levels
- Promotes digestion and stomach health
- Aids blood circulation
- Aids weight loss
- Good for heart health
- Relieves joint pain
- Anti-cancerous

Now out of all these great effects, form the point of view of gut health we are interested in ACV because of its Ph. balancing effects and also because of its effects on balancing stomach health.

There are two factors worth considering here. Firstly, ACV helps to balance the acidic levels within the stomach. Acid reflux is seen as an imbalance in the stomach, whereby acid spurts up from the stomach into the oesophagus thus creating heart burn. However, from a holistic point of view, acid reflux is not caused by erratic acid activity, but rather it is caused by insufficient stomach acid levels. Where ACV helps is that it balances the Ph. environment in the stomach, thus helping to normalise stomach acidic activity. So even though ACV, like wheatgrass acts as a base on the body, however ACV is actually an acid, so while it converts into a base after digestion, prior to digestion it is acidic and it helps the stomach balance its acid levels!

The second advantage is that it works while promoting an acidic environment in the stomach which encourages lactobacilli, which are helpful bacteria which thrive in an acidic environment and help to maintain a healthy gut and help to kill off gut fungi such as Candida!

ACV is very easy to take, simply take one tablespoon of ACV in a glass and add in 250ml (8ounces) of water, stir with a spoon and drink. The only thing to watch out for with ACV is that it is acidic, so make sure you wash your teeth by rinsing your mouth out with some water or another beverage afterwards, so as to wash away the acidic deposits from the teeth. Other than that ACV is easy to take although it is bitter in taste. Also the ideal ACV is slightly smoky in colour because it possesses a string of material known as 'the mother' which is very potent. So when buying ACV try and get the version of ACV which is a little bit misty in colour.

ACV will have a general balancing effect on gut health and is really helpful for people who suffer with acid reflux problems. However, it's not the sort of supplement which you take when you have acute acid reflux symptoms. When you are suffering from acid reflux and you want to treat the symptom take an antacid, natural yoghurt or milk. But get into the habit of taking at least one glass a day of ACV and over a period of a few weeks it will have an impact on stomach acid and gut health in general.

Also ACV goes really well with wheatgrass. I find that washing down a glass of ACV with a glass of wheatgrass is a good way to get my daily quota of both and of course the wheatgrass washes of the acidic ACV deposits form my teeth as wheatgrass is a base.

Kombucha

Kombucha is a popular health drink, which is basically a sugary black tea, which after fermentation it becomes laden with healthy bacteria, vinegar, b vitamins, probiotics, enzymes and healthy acids (acetic, lactic and gluconic).

Benefits of kombucha includes:

- Gut health
- Weight loss
- Detoxification
- Improved immune system
- Reduced joint pain
- Anti-cancerous

In particular, from the point of view of gut health the really great thing about kombucha is its amazing variety of probiotics which help to keep the digestive process working properly.

Kombucha is high in Acetobacter , Gluconacetobacte, Lactobacillus and Zygosaccharomyces probiotics. So kombucha will go along way towards getting your gut to work well. With so many probiotics these will flush out funguses (such as Candida) and aid in digestion.

43

Also kombucha is high in free antioxidants, which helps to counteract free radicals in the gut, which also aids digestive health. Kombucha has also been known to treat stomach ulcers and helps both to prevent and treat leaky gut syndrome.

Kombucha is a very powerful gut health tonic and one or two glasses a day, will go along way towards improving stomach and gut health. But do note that there are so many probiotics in kombucha that if your gut is out of balance, that initially kombucha might result in symptoms such as bloatedness, gas, mild stomach ache and diarrhoea. Don't' worry about this, as it is the guts way of normalising under the powerful and potent impact of kombucha. So when you start taking kombuhca, ease into it by taking one glass a day for a few days and then build up to two or three glasses a day, then after a few weeks when you feel things settle down, then reduce back to a maintenance level, of one glass a day.

Kefir: Kefir is a
Turkish cultured dairy product, which is very high in probiotics. Kefir has been used as a health food for centuries and amongst its many benefits are:

- Improves immunity levels
- Heals gut problems
- Helps digest lactose
- Kills of Candida fungus
- Treats allergies
- Strengthens bones
- Detoxicant

44

Kefir's many benefits come from its nutrient rich make-up. Kefir is high in vitamin B12, vitamin K2, calcium, biotin, folate, probiotics and enzymes. In particular enzymes and probiotics make kefir a very potent gut health food.

Enzymes reduce once one reaches 30 years of age, which in turn makes it more difficult to digest food, so eating a supplement which is high in digestive enzymes is a great way of improving digestion. Secondly probiotics are healthy bacteria and healthy bacteria fight of nasty digestive fungus's such as Candida, for example.

Kefir is jam packed with probiotics which includes Bifidobacteria, Acetobacter, Lactobacillus Acidophilus, Lactobacillus Bulgaricus, Lactobacillus Caucasus, Lactobacillus Rhamnosus, Lactobacillus and Leuconostoc.

The result of this is that kefir can heal many gut issues include Leaky Gut Syndrome. Also, interestingly it helps people who suffer from lactose intolerance to actually start absorbing lactose!

For anyone who is suffering from gut health issues kefir is worth trying out. However, kefir being a dairy product, it might be difficult to take for anyone who is lactose intolerant. People who suffer with Candida, for example, are lactose intolerant, so they won't initially be able to absorb kefir. In this case it makes more sense to make an effort to detoxify and clean up the digestive system in the first place. So take other supplements such as wheatgrass, ACV and ginger for a while and then slowly add in the kefir.

Moringa

Moringa is a tree which grows well in Southeast Asia, and is often referred to as the "miracle tree" because it is very high in nutrients which includes beta carotene, Vitamin C, carotene and protein.

Moringa is so high in nutrients that it has 12 times more vitamin C than an oranges, it has 10 times more vitamin A than carrots and 17 times more calcium than milk, for example!

From the point of view of gut health moringa can help in several ways. For a start moringa is high in antioxidants, which helps to detox the intestines. Secondly, moringa helps to reduce inflammation in the body. Inflammation is the body's way of coping with imbalances in the body; it's a sort of cordon whereby the body cordons off infected areas. For a short time it works well, but after a while chronic health develops. Inflammation in the gut is a real bad thing, as it makes food nutrients absorption difficult and also excretion of wastes difficult. So morninga can help to reduce inflammation through the body, which includes the gut. Also moringa boosts liver functioning, which helps to detoxify the system, which is good as where there is a dysfunctional gut, there will be a buildup of toxins in the body.

46

Moringa leafs can be used with your meals as in a salad or in a juice, for example. If you cannot get your hands on raw moringa, you can probable get a hold of organic cold – pressed moringa oil. Moringa oil is expensive, but it's potent with about a tablespoonful a day being a really good overall health tonic and of course a gut treatment for gut health problems.

Supplements for Gut Health

So far we have looked at foods which help to cure gut health problems, but there are also some supplements which can help, so let's take a look.

Deglycyrrhizinated licorice (DGL)

Licorice is very good for health and helps cure or improve a wide range of health conditions. However, long-term usage can have a negative impact upon blood pressure levels, oedema and oestrogen levels, thanks to the presence of glycyrrhizin. Whereas deglycyrrhizinated licorice, has all the benefits of licorice but without the potential downsides of glycyrrhizin.

From the point of view of gut health, DGL provides great relief for heartburn, peptic ulcers and gastritis, which relates back to its anti-inflammatory properties and its gut bacteria balancing properties. In a study of 82 patients who took DGL, versus an over the counter peptic ulcer medication, the patients who were

47

given 2 DGL tablets daily, over a period of two years, demonstrated the same level of reoccurrence of peptic ulcers, as the patients who took the peptic ulcer medicine, which suggests that DGL is just as strong as the allopathic medication! 4

They also note noted in this study that the DGL group, just like the pharmaceutical group, suffered from a big increase in the onset of peptic ulcers after they stopped taking DGL. This suggests that while DGL is as effective as pharmaceutical medications at treating peptic ulcers, it only keeps peptic ulcers at bay, as long as it was taken. So for some people who suffer extreme stomach issues, such as peptic ulcers, DGL will probably end up becoming part of a lifelong treatment plan!

Regarding dosage, usually DGL is taken anywhere from 1 to 3 tablets, at a dosage of 380 to 400mg per tablet. Take the DGL tablet about 30 minutes prior to each meal will help relieve your stomach.

With that in mind, it's important to remember that long-term herbal supplement use can have toxic side effects, just like long-term medications can. With DGL, the majority of the glycyrrhizin has been removed, however, a little still remains, so if you decide to use DGL, over a long period of time, do check your blood pressure, from time to time, and watch out for oedema. Also in some cases liver toxicity can occur. Dglycyrrhizinated licorice, is a great supplement and chances are that there will be no side effects, but this is something to bear in mind for anyone who is on long term medication, and DGL been just as effective as a pharmaceutical drug should be respected as potentially damaging to health, in some cases.

As to why you should use DGL rather than using pharmaceutical drugs, DGL being a natural product will have less side effects, but like any powerful herb, some toxic side effects shall still remain present.

And this is something to remember with the various foods, supplements and health tips mentioned in this book. In an ideal world every health condition would be curable, but in reality gut health can vary from individual to individual. For some people, they will get great relief from their symptoms with a few small changes. Anyone who suffers from a strong food allergy can testify to this! However, for some people no matter how many strategies they try, or foods they take, their gut health issues linger on. For people in this group, the thing to remember is that gut health is a complex topic and although a full-blown cure may not come, certainly with patience and application of good healing strategies, foods and supplements, much relief can be achieved.

So if you have tried everything under the sun and yet still suffer with gut health issues don't despair. Things will get better, but some trial and error may be required, and even if a full recovery does not come, certainly a good improvement can be made. The reason for writing this book is to share some resources with you, which you might not have already considered. While modern health care can help in many ways, there is a tendency to treat patients symptomatically by providing different drugs to treat various symptoms. I'm not saying that complementary health care is better, but what I am saying is that it provides us with some more resources and other options and also that it focuses upon balance, where a rebalance can take place often symptoms will take care of themselves!

Betaine Hydrochloric Acid

Betaine Hydrochoric Acid is an ideal supplement for people who are suffering from insufficient stomach acid levels. As noted earlier from a complementary point of view, acid reflux is as a direct consequence of deficient stomach acid levels, which result in sporadic production of hydrochloric acid in the stomach, some of which ends up in the oesophagus which results in acid reflux symptoms. Apple Cider Vinegar can help to restore this balance as ACV is an acid, but for more severe cases if ACV doesn't appear to help, it's worth trying out Betaine Hydrochloric Acid.

Betaine HCL will help to rebalance the acid levels in the stomach, which will not only cures acid reflux, but also it help to improve the overall health and vitality of the stomach and gut and finally sufficient levels of HCL are required to effectively breakdown and digest vitamin B12, amino acids and proteins!

Regarding dosage a little bit of trial and error is required. Start by taking a meal which contains at least 20 grams of protein (HCL is required to breakdown the protein). Take 1 Betaine HCL pills (around 650mg) and check in with your stomach, after eating, to see if it has made any difference to digestion. You should feel better, but if you feel a burning sensation chances are that too much acid is been taking. If you feel a burning distension feeling, then reduce down to

50

half a pill. If you feel an improvement or don't feel any improvement, just maintain this one pill per meal and after a couple of days try out 2 pills and see how you feel. Keep experimenting with dosage until you feel an improvement in digestion, but don't feel any discomfort. Once you feel discomfort stop and even reduce dosage a little bit, if need be.

So experiment a little bit, until you are taking enough Betaine HCL, to make a good improvement to digestion, without overdoing it as too much HCL will make you feel ill. For most people the dosing of Betaine HCL shall be somewhere between 3000mg to 5500mg per meal. Taking too little won't do anything to help digestion and taking too much will make for an over acidic gut environment.

Contraindications

One thing which you have to be careful about, when using Betaine HCL, and that is when Betaine HCL is mixed with anti-inflammatory drugs such as aspirin, corticosteroids, Indocin, ibuprofen and NSAIDs (non-steroidal anti-inflammatory drug) in general. The reason is that HCL pills, when mixed into a stomach, which is already containing these drugs can aggravate the stomach lining and even result in bleeding of the stomach lining, or even the development of an ulcer!

So while Betaine HCL is a great way to improve acid reflux and indigestion, you have to be careful otherwise you can make things worse!

Also, anti-inflammatory drugs are very popular, ibuprofen for example (Motrin, Advil, Brofen) is a very popular headache pill, and of course aspirin is very popular, so just check out your medications and don't mix these medications with HCL!

L-glutamine

L-Glutamine is a very useful supplement. L-Glutamine is an amino acid, being the most common amino acid used by the human body (around 30 present of all amino acid nitrogen in the blood is L-Glutamine). Being an amino acid, L-Glutamine will obviously be a big help at building muscle and maintaining lean muscle when dieting, but it also comes with many other benefits which includes:

- L-Glutamine is great for intestinal health, as it helps to rebuild and repair damage to the gut
- It helps to heal ulcers, cure leaky gut syndrome and prevents further damage to the stomach and intestines
- It improves symptoms of Irritable Bowel Syndrome (IBS) and diarrhoea by balancing mucus levels in the stomach lining.5
- Reduces cravings for sweets and alcohol
- Improves the metabolism
- Detoxifies the body (including the intestines)
- Improves blood sugar control

52

- Anti-cancer agent
- Promotes muscle growth and prevents muscle wasting
- Improves athletic performance and recovery from exercise

So in essence L-Glutamine is a body builder, which in the case of gut issues, it is a body rebuilder, helping to repair gut health issues.

In a study of 20 patients who were fed intravenously for two weeks, they noted that the group, who received L-Glutamine, along with the intravenous food, suffered less gastrointestinal degeneration and demonstrated better permeability than those who didn't. Intravenous feeding has a negative impact upon digestive health, so this study demonstrates the potency of L-Glutamine.6

In another study they noted the healing mechanism of L-Glutamine, whereby it regulates the IgA immune response. IgA is an antibody which fights against bad bacteria and viruses. It also relates to food sensitivities and allergies. So take L-Glutamine will help with food intolerances.7

In yet another study in the Journal of Clinical Immunology they discovered that L-Glutamine regulates the TH2 immune response, which in turn regulates inflammatory cytokines.8 so what this means is that L-Glutamine reduces inflammatory responses, which in turn helps to reduce many gut imbalances.

In summary L-Glutamine can repair damage, reduce food sensitivity and allergic responses and also reduce or even eliminate the inflammatory effect.

L-Glutamine is a must have supplement, for anyone who is facing gut repair issues. Leaky Gut syndrome, for example, isn't just uncomfortable but rather it promotes other degenerative health conditions, such as autoimmune conditions, psoriasis, arthritis and even Hashimotos' disease (a slow thyroid).

When we think about healing gut issues, we have to think in terms of getting rid of toxins, righting imbalances and also repairing organic damage and this is where L-Glutamine comes in handy.

L-Glutamine helps with repairing damage caused by a wide variety of gut health issues including Chrohn's disease, Irritable Bowel Syndrome (IBS), Ulcerative colitis, Diverticulosis and Diverticulitis, for example.

How to Take L-Glutamine

L-Glutamine comes in two forms, which are free form, which has to be taken with food for proper absorption. The other type is known as Trans-Alanyl Glutamine or Alanyl –L - Glutamine. This latter time is more absorbable that free form L-GLutmine, so you can take it on an empty stomach, if you want to. You can take it after your meals and in particular it is helpful either before or

54

after workouts in the gym, as it supports both athletic performance and repair of muscle damage.

Regarding dosage, dosage is usually 2 to 5 grams a day, but up to 10 grams a day can be taken. For people with gut health, it makes most sense to take it three times a day, during mealtime either just before or just after food, so as to help with the digestive process. Also for long-term use it is a good idea to supplement some vitamin B12 every day, which helps to regulate L-Glutamine levels in the body, a sot much L-0Glutamine can result in some toxicity, if too much builds up in the body.

Side effects of too much L-Glutamine includes increased sweating in feet and hands, back pain, joint pain, muscle pain, dizziness, fatigue, headache, runny nose, dry mouth, gas, vomiting and stomach pain. These are unlikely to happen but it's good to know. The vitamin B12 should minimize the tendency of side effects, but if some of these symptoms arise, then reduces dosage accordingly.

Contraindications: L-Glutamine should be avoided for people who are suffering with liver or kidney dysfunction.

Aloe Vera

Aloe Vera is a super plant which has many great benefits which includes:

55

- High in anti-inflammatory properties

- Helps relieve constipation

- Promotes regular bowel movements

- Detoxification

- Encourages good gut bacteria

- Helps treat leaky gut syndrome

- Helps relieve heartburn/acid reflux

- High in antioxidant and antibacterial properties

- Fights off candida fungus

- Fights off parasitic infections

- Treats mouth ulcers

- Reduces dental plaque

- Improves skin quality

- Prevents wrinkles

So in summary aloe Vera is an amazing plant which demonstrates a wide range of effects. In particular it works wonderfully well on gut health.

Aloe Vera is high in nutrients including calcium, copper, chromium, magnesium, manganese, potassium, sodium, selenium and zinc; It is high in the antioxidant vitamins A, C and E; it is also a great source of vitamin B12, choline and folic acid. Furthermore, aloe Vera contains 8 digestive enzymes (alianase, amylase, alkaline phosphatase, catalase, carboxypeptidase, cellulose, lipase and peroxidase) which help to break down foods. Also, Aloe Vera is high in probiotics (healthy gut bacteria), which help to restore the balance of gut health. In a study on the effect of Aloe Vera on lactobacilli probiotics, they noted a significant increase in levels of L. acidophilus, L. plantarum and L. casei, via aloe vera supplementation.8 Finally Aloe Vera promotes regulation of Ph. Levels throughout the body, which in turn aids gut health.

How to Take Aloe Vera

There is a variety of ways in which you can take aloe Vera. You can take it as a juice or as a capsule. Regarding dosage you can start on a small amount, say 1tsp twice a day taken before meals. Then slowly increase the amount taken up to a maximum of 4 tbsp. twice a day. How much you will take, will vary according to your gut health issues and your reaction to aloe Vera juice or capsules. Aloe Vera promotes bowel movements, so it is a good idea to start of, taken a small amount particularly at first, since it will help to clear any backlog within the intestines, hence too much too soon might result in diarrhoea like symptoms!

Also on the other hand many people avoid aloe Vera, believing it to be a laxative, but actually it is quite safe to take and even kids can take it, but they should take a very small l amount like a tsp. or two per day. Rather aloe Vera is safe but it does rebalance bowel movements and can result in a laxative like effect, if you take too much too soon!

Footnotes

1. Ginger for Nausea and Vomiting in Pregnancy: Randomized, Double-Masked, Placebo-Controlled Trial

    VUTYAVANICH, TERAPORN MD, MSC;
    KRAISARIN, THEERAJANA MD;
    RUANGSRI, RUNG-AROON BSC.

2. Eur J Gastroenterol Hepatol. 2008 May;20(5):436-40. doi: 10.1097/MEG.0b013e3282f4b224.

    Effects of ginger on gastric emptying and motility in healthy humans.

    Wu KL[1], Rayner CK, Chuah SK, Changchien CS, Lu SN, Chiu YC, Chiu KW, Lee CM.

    [1]Division of Hepatogastroenterology, Department of Internal Medicine, College of Medicine, Chang Gung Memorial Hospital, Kaohsiung Medical Center, Chang Gung University, Kaohsiung, Taiwan. kengliang_wu@yahoo.com.tw

3. Peppermint oil: a treatment for postoperative nausea
    Sylvina Tate MSc BSc (Hons) RGN DipN PGDE RNT*
    Article first published online: 28 JUN 2008

DOI: 10.1046/j.1365-2648.1997.t01-15-00999.x

4. Morgan AG, Pacsoo C, McAdam WA (June 1985). "Maintenance therapy: a two year comparison between Caved-S and cimetidine treatment in the prevention of symptomatic gastric ulcer recurrence." Gut 26 (6): 599-602.

5. HIV Clin Trials. 2003 Sep-Oct;4(5):324-9.

L-glutamine supplementation improves nelfinavir-associated diarrhea in HIV-infected individuals.

Huffman FG[1], Walgren ME.

[1]Department of Dietetics and Nutrition, College of Health and Urban Affairs, Florida International University, Miami, Florida 33172, USA. huffmanf@fiu.edu

6. Glutamine and the preservation of gut integrity
R.R.W.J. van der Hulst MD, M.F. von Meyenfeldt MD, N.E.P. Deutz MD, P.B. Soeters MD (Prof), R.J.M. Brummer MD, B.K. von Kreel PhD, J.W. Arends MD (Prof)
Published: 29 May 1993

7. Clin Immunol. 1999 Dec;93(3):294-301.

Effect of glutamine on Th1 and Th2 cytokine responses of human peripheral blood mononuclear cells.

Chang WK[1], Yang KD, Shaio MF.

8. Gut Microbes. 2012 Jan 1; 3(1): 4–14.

doi: 10.4161/gmic.19320

PMCID: PMC3337124

The role of gut microbiota in immune homeostasis and autoimmunity

Hsin-Jung Wu [1,2,*] and Eric Wu

9. Acta Biomed. 2012 Dec;83(3):183-8.

Effect of Aloe vera juice on growth and activities of Lactobacilli in-vitro.

Nagpal R[1], Kaur V, Kumar M, Marotta F.

We are human beings and this means that we are living in physical bodies and these bodies are a handy way of getting around and living our lives!

So there is a tendency to take our bodies for granted and never a truer word has been said! Often due to a sedentary lifestyle and a lifestyle whereby we sit all day, our bodies become unbalanced and we need to regain our balance to improve our health and this includes our acid reflux!

Deep breathing for Acid Reflux Presentation and Relief

In a 2011 study of the Journal of Gastroentology1 noted how deep breathing exercises could help to both prevent and reduce symptoms of acid reflux by strengthening the diaphragm which in turn strengthens the oesophageal sphincter (a small round muscles which opens and closes – if it's weak acid will easily cross over from the stomach into the oesophagus).

When the lower oesophageal sphincter (LES) muscle becomes weak it encourages acid reflux events, so by using deep breathing exercises we strengthen the LES and within days a significant reduction in acid reflux will take place!

How to Perform Deep breathing for Acid Reflux

1.   Simply lie down, breathe out and then breathe in deeply into your belly.

2. Keep on breathing into your lower belly as if you were filling a balloon until it feels fairly full.

3. Hold for a second and then breath out and keep on breathing out until you have to squeeze your abdominal muscles a little bit, hold for a second.

4. Then repeat 10 times.

5. Take a 10 second break and then repeat again twice.

This exercise will do a lot to help with your LES, but also it will help to strengthen your abs and core muscles, it will help to regenerate your stomach lining, it will help to massage your lower intestines which in turn will help with digestion, fighting nutritional deficiencies and generally boosting overall health and wellbeing, as well as help out with acid reflux!

Marjariasana (Cat Asana) & Bitilasana (Cow Pose)

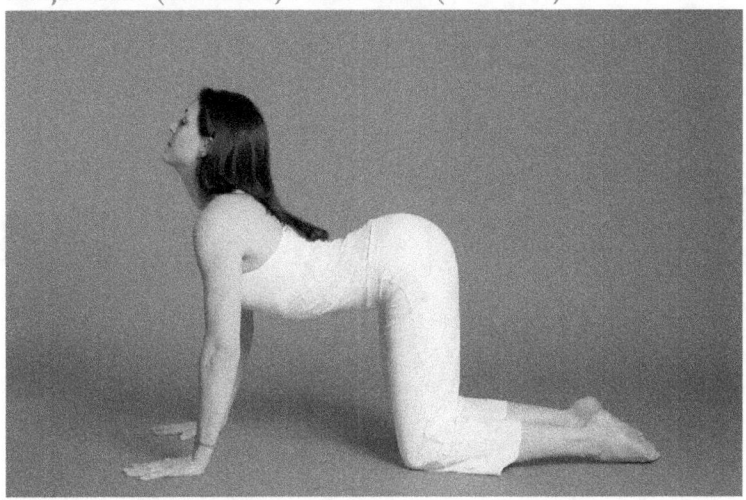

Bitilasana is a great exercise for working the posture, hips, spine and digestive organs and it works great in tandem with the cat asana.

Directions:

1. Sit on all fours, so that your back forms a table top and your feet and hands form the legs.

2. The knees should be placed under your hips, and your wrists should be in the same line as your shoulders.

3. Let your head droop in a neutral position. Gaze softly in the direction of the floor.

4. Inhale, and lift your buttocks up while at the same time as lifting your chest. Let your abdomen drop towards the ground, while you lift your head and look forward or upwards.

63

5. Hold this pose for a few seconds, then, breathe out and come back to the tabletop position.

MARJARIASANA

Inhale, & come into cow pose

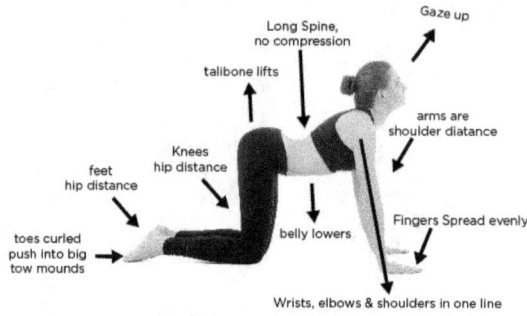

Exhale & come into cat pose

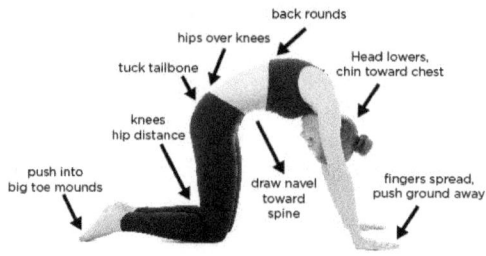

It works the core muscles and benefits the digestive organs and the spine.

Directions:

1. Sit on all fours, so that your back forms a table top and your feet and hands form the legs.

2. Arms should be perpendicular to the floor, and hands should be placed flat on the floor, under the shoulders. Knees should be placed hip-width apart.

3. Looking straight ahead, inhale and lower your chin as you tilt your head in a forwards direction, while pulling your belly upwards and raising your bottom at the same time, and finish of by squeezing your bottom. Compress your buttocks.

5. Hold the pose for a few breaths and breathe deeply.

6. Now use the following countermovement: As you exhale, lower your chin to your chest while arching your back up as much as you can.

6. Do these two movements(cat and cow) about five to six times.

Adho mukha śvānāsana (downward-facing dog Pose)

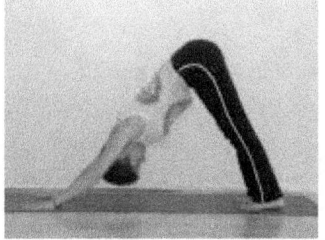

Picture courtesy of wikipedia

Downward facing dog is an all round body builder. It particularly developes the trapezius muscles of the upper back, the latissimus dorsi (outer back muscles), the back of the arms (tricpes), the bottom (gluteus maximus) and the back of the thighs (hamstrings). It also has a secondary effect on the mid back (rhomboids), the primary shoulder tendons (rotator cuff), the front and side shoulder muscles (anterior and medial deltoids), the rear shoulder muscles (posterior deltoids) the muscles of the lower side of the body (serratus), and the calf muscles (soleus and gastrocnemius).

Now where this exercise helps the rehab and prehab of back pain is because it tones up all the muscles of the posterior chain and it also tighten the core muscles of the midsection. It tightens up the abdomen and the lower back muscles and the side muscles (the serratus), which make the physique more stable and grounded thus healing old injuries and preventing new ones from taking place.

To perform this exercise simply lie down with your face touching the floor and your hands palm downwards parallel to your face. Now lift your bottom and hips up from the floor while pushing up both with the heels of your feet and your hands pushing upwards so that your body will now resemble a roof with feet and hands at opposite ends and your bottom at the peak postion.

Now ideally you should stay in this position for between 20 to 25 breaths, which could be very taxing at the early stages. More importantly when in this peak position try to focus on breathing in and out steadily and feeling the energy movemetn with the body. Try and feel the exercises, feel your breaht, feel the energy flow and the tension in the muscles. If you can only stay in this position for a few breaths then fine you will increase over time!

Bālāsana (Child's Resting Pose)

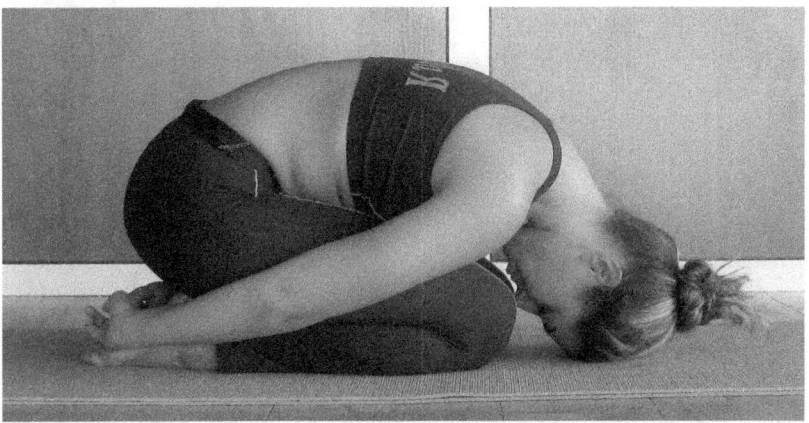

Picture courtesy of wikipedia

After performing downward facing dog the relaxed poise to follow straight afterwards is the child's resting pose. It's fairly straight forward to oerform. Simply sit down on your knees and let your torso lay down on your thighs and your head on the floor or as near to the floor as possible. Also you have to let your arms droop and relax while holding your hands over your heels.

Now for many of us this is a tough pose to perform correctly as we tend to be so stiff that it's difficult to reach the floor with our heads and even our torso's get stuck halfway down with our shoulders and heads been way of the floor. However, with practice the position will become easier to perform. The key is absolute relaxation of the back muscles and this is also why this exercise combines so well with downward dog because we have just drilled our back muscles and now we give them complete rest. Try and feel the muscles of your mid back and simply let them stretch and relax, as they do so your torso and head will dropp down.

This exercise is a really great way to take stress out of your back and also its really good for spinal health and general rest and relaxation!

ARDHA MATSYENDRASANA (Half Spinal Twist Pose)

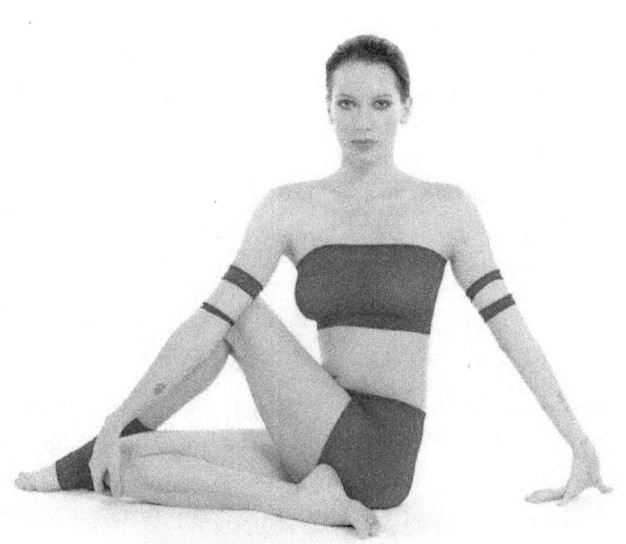

Picture courtesy of wikipedia user Kennguru

alexey baykov http://yogashaktipat.com yoga.shaktipat@gmail..com

This is a great poise for working on stretching the latsissimus dorsi muslces of the back (the outer back muscles). Also it creates a stretch from the hips right through the width of the back and right up into the beck which gives the entire back area a good stretch. In particular while stretching the nerves which run along the spine are stimualted with fresh blood and so too are the ligaments and tendons. This exercise is good for both rehab and prehab and if practised regularly it will go a long way towards ensuring back health.

It's a little ticky to get it right at first as the pose feels counter intuitive. Basicaly you are going to sit with your left leg crossed over your folded right knee and then holding the right knee with your right hand while reaching around almost towards your back with your left hand and then pulling the spine into a gentle twist. Hold the position until you feel a good stretch and take a few breaths. Release and then do again three more times. Then swap over this time you will be turning your torso to the right hand side and placing your reight leg over your folded left knee, repeat four times in total!

One foot is placed flat on the floor outside the opposite leg and torso twists toward the top leg. The bottom leg may be bent with the foot outside the opposite hip, or extended with toes vertical. The arms help leverage the torso into the twist and may be bound (Baddha Ardha Matsyendrasana) in a number of configurations by clutching either feet or opposite hands.

Traditional Chinese Medicine and Oriental Energetic Exercises

Tradional Chinese Medicine (TCM) can go a long way towards balancing the various channels in the bodya dn the energetic organs which connect them. For example, if the stomach channel is in excess acid reflux will kick off. TCM is a very complex subject and interestingly two people could have the same . symptoms but with different aetiologies. The best approach then is to seek out a TCM practitioner or acupuncturist of good repute and get them to treat you on a regular basis.

TCM and acupuncture are not miracle workers but often regular treatment over a period of months will go a long way towards relieving symptoms of acid reflux and rebuilding the health balance required so that a long-term cure can eventually take place. While this book attempts to provide you with some practical self-help points, seeking a professional acupuncturist or other complementary health practitioner can be a really good idea. And it's not restricted to Chinese medicine, as while Chine medicine is good, many people have also receive a great result from Ayurveda medicine and homeopathy also!

The best approach to take is not to get too attached to results. One person might go to an acupuncturist and make no progress, but then they go to another complementary healer and they get a cure and yet it can just as easily work the other way to. So why is it that these therapies seem to vary in their effectiveness?

This is a really good question, but the answer is rather difficult, in that each human being is complex and so what works for one may not work for another.

I also have a pet theory that often when a person gets a cure using a particular therapy, that it's not that this therapy is better than other therapies but rather that over a period of months or even years this person is trying really hard to rebalance their body and as a result of this finally the body finds this balance. Of course humans being what they are they tend to hail the health system which cured them, as the best, when in fact really they cured themselves by taking a sensible approach to their treatment!

Oriental Energetic Systems

Oriental energetic systems such as Tai Chi and Qi Gong work quite effectively and indeed they work the same way as hatha yoga, with the difference been that they are easier to perform, for they are very gentle movements and do not require much in the way of flexibility or physical exuberance. On the downside though in some ways hatha yoga can stimulate the body in a more intense way.

Take a look at the three exercises below, they may or may not directly help relieve your stomach acidity problems, but either way they will greatly enhance true overall strength and wellbeing of the body and in the process of reinforcing the subtle energies of the body, often it will help to reduce or even cure acid reflux symptoms along the way. And this is a very important point, for curing acid reflux is not about a quick fix, rather it's about creating a foundation of balance within the body and then finishing off with some practical everyday strategies. The exercises below are not everyday strategies to treat acid reflux symptoms, but they are a foundation which will encourage the strengthening of the subtle inner body (etheric body) and thus over time these exercises will go a long way towards improving overall health levels!

The Crane, The Turtle and the Solar Plexus Exercises

If you Google these exercises, a few options will come up and most of them are difficult to perform. However, exercises of the same name but which are easy to perform, and at the same time are very beneficial, have already been popularised back in the early 1980's by Stephen T Chang and his famous books on Taoist healing techniques. I like these particular variations because of their simplicity and effectiveness. There are lots of interesting exercises, out there, but which are difficult to perform, and really it's not necessary to wrap your legs around your head, in order to heal your body. Rather, many exercises which originate from taoist healing systems, are very easy to perform and should be popularised once again because they really are that good.

Crane

Starting with the Crane, it is named in deference to the crane bird which sucks its abdomen in towards its back bone when standing. A simple variation of this is to simply lie on your back and breath. Breath out while trying to suck your navel back in towards your spine, then breath in and literarily fill up your abdomen until it bloats outward, almost as if it's about to burst. Sucking ones abdomen inwards massages the stomach and intestines, while breathing very deeply into the abdomen charges the stomach with air. Young babies practice abdominal breathing, whilst most adults perform superficial breathing via the top of their lungs, breathing from the abdomen is the natural way to breath. Filling the abdomen first and then the lungs results in a really deep and beneficial breath.

Benefits

The crane has several benefits, which includes the following:

- Strengthening the stomach (which aids digestion and energy production)
- Massaging the intestines (which aids digestion and energy production and prevents constipation)
- Deep breathing stimulates the nervous system and oxygenates the blood (which in turn reduces blood pressure)
- Deep breathing combined with deep exhalations extract toxins from the blood
- Deep inhalations combined with deep exhalations, carried out with conscious intent promotes yang energy (active energy) in the body.

Technique

1. Lie down.
2. Breath out, while sucking in your abdomen, focus upon the navel retracting towards the spinal cord. Go as far as is comfortable and then squeeze slightly. This process can then be enhanced by pressing gently downwards, with the palms of your hands.
3. When fully exhaled immediately inhale, by breathing into the abdomen and filling up your belly until it fills like its ready to explode. At this stage the breath will naturally fill the lungs from the lower position. Hold for a few seconds and then exhale once again.

4. Repeat this process of exhalation followed by deep inhalation and continue for about five minutes in total.

It is important, with this exercise to carry it out gently. Do not force, rather gently exhale and gently inhale. Also, there is a good chance that some slight discomfort will be felt during the exhalation. This is fine, the reason for this, is because most of us have backed up faeces, within our intestines. Which is a common, side effect of highly processed foods, and lack of fibre in our diet. Keep with the program and gently massage the lower intestines, by gently squeezing (but not forcing) the lower intestines.

With this exercise, blood will gently seep into the microvilli of the lower intestines, which in turn will aid digestion and health in general.

What has this exercise got to do with high blood pressure?

This is a great exercise for building up the two most important organs of the body, from the point of view of health and vitality. A strong stomach will break down food efficiently, while strong clean intestines will effectively absorb nutrients into the body. The effect of these two organs been boosted is an improved immune system, higher vitality levels and improved yang (active) energy, which in turn helps to balance blood pressure naturally.

The Solar Plexus Exercise

Like Stephen T Chang, I am a great believer in this exercise, although the way I do it differs considerable from his method. The way I recommend doing this exercise is twofold, it involves massaging the solar plexus and also using visualisation exercises.

From a nervous point of view, the solar plexus is a major nerve group, within the body. The solar plexus is found at the base of the sternum. Lie down and poke this area with your finger, when a sudden stabbing pain is felt, then bingo!..this is the solar plexus. From a TCM point of view, the solar plexus represents the emotional brain, while the physical brain is simply a computing machine. Whenever we feel upset or overwhelmed, we feel discomfort in the solar plexus. Stage nerves, when we have to step up and speak in front of others and feeling nauseous when facing an interview, are obvious examples of an overwhelmed solar plexus. Also, in the case of kids, often their stomach aches are actually caused by emotional overwhelming feelings, in the solar plexus and massaging will often help greatly.

The solar plexus is really important, because our bodies are designed for a far more simple era, consequently, we often feel overwhelmed because we are designed for simple living.

Solar plexus exercises, will greatly help to calm down anxious feelings and obviously this will help blood pressure levels because of the feelings of rejuvenation which come from this exercise, since often high blood pressure levels are created by tension and feelings of being overwhelmed. So this is a great deep relaxation exercise.

Technique

1. Lie down.
2. Locate the solar plexus and begin massaging it in a clockwise manner. This is particularly useful when feeling hurt feelings and anxious feelings. If general fatigue is felt, but emotions are not disturbed then just jump ahead to the next stage.
3. Hold both hands either side of the solar plexus and then visualise divine white light (or egg yolk yellow, if you like – as this is the astral colour of the solar plexus chakra) gently filling the solar plexus.
4. Maintain this position and occasionally remind oneself of the light. Continue for five to fifteen minutes.

Also, if you like soft music can be played along while this gently recharging process is taking place.

Turtle

The turtle is a simple exercise, yet it is a great way to relax the neck and shoulders, which in turn brings about relaxation and consequently this de-stressing effect promotes relief of high blood pressure.

Benefits

1. Stretches the spine.
2. Relaxes the shoulders and neck.
3. Boosts the thyroid and parathyroid.
4. Boosts the metabolism.
5. Boosts inner energy delivery within the body.

Technique

1. Sit (cross legged or on a chair).
2. Bring your chin down to your chest and slowly inhale. The neck will feel slightly stretched while the shoulders will relax deeply.
3. Slowly lift the head upwards and backwards, until the back of the head touched the atlas joint, at the back of the neck. Exhale while doing so, this time the throat will feel stretched.

4.   Repeat twelve times, but do not strain.

Contraindications

In general this is a very safe exercise but do bear in mind that for someone who suffers from serious neck injuries or scoliosis, for example, might feel pain and it might be damaging. So obviously, use your common sense. No discomfit should be felt either during or after this exercise. If any discomfort if felt, do stop immediately!

Footnotes

1.   Am J Gastroenterol. 2012 Mar;107(3):372-8. doi: 10.1038/ajg.2011.420. Epub 2011 Dec 6.

Positive effect of abdominal breathing exercise on gastroesophageal reflux disease: a randomized, controlled study.

Eherer AJ[1], Netolitzky F, Högenauer C, Puschnig G, Hinterleitner TA, Scheidl S, Kraxner W, Krejs GJ, Hoffmann KM.

In this book we have covered quite a wide range of strategies for curing acid reflux, which includes lifestyle, dietary/supplements and exercise related. So putting it all together what is the best policy regarding curing yourself of acid reflux?

The first thing to realise is that allopathic medicine doesn't have a good understanding of what is causing acid reflux and if it did then a cure would surely have come around by now. I don't mean to criticise but from my experience as a TCM practitioner, acid reflux is treated by prescription drugs only, from a western medical point of view. Tests are taken and it appears severe and speeches are made about lifestyle and genetics, meanwhile the gastrointestinal world looks forward to the next major chemical leap forward towards treating (notice treating not curing) acid reflux. Also they have a tendency to label things, so if you suffer from frequent bouts of acid reflux they label it as GERD, but other than a label does this help you, and if it's a 'disease' than what about an aetiology and a cure?

The reason why allopathic medicine is not good at curing conditions like acid reflux is because they tend to treat the body like a bunch of LEGO pieces, treating one body part as if it where complete unrelated to the others. In reality everything is interrelated and in particular a very complex and large series of organs (which the gastrointestinal tract is) represents a very potentially complex set of possibilities which could all be working, one way or another, towards bringing on acid reflux.

So if you want a cure, then think in terms of balancing your body and in particular long-term imbalances take a long time to cure. If say, for example, you have been suffering from acid reflux symptoms for one year and no other symptoms before this, then sure you might cure it in a week or two, but if you have had acid reflux symptoms for a year a and a build-up of lots of other gastrointestinal disturbances, over say the last decade, it might take months to make an impact and a year or two to really correct the problem!

So be patient and think in terms of balance.

Another factor to consider also is the difference between treatment and cure. In the long-term we need cure, but often in the short-term we need treatment. The person who is suffering from migraine problems might take months before they are cured, but are they going to wait for months to cure a single headache? I think not! So if say you have a bout of acid reflux today, then you have to follow some tactics to treat it. This can be natural cures and supplements, but of course it can also be over the counter or prescription antacids. I'm not against pharmaceutical drugs they have their place, it's just that they won't cure your acid reflex as their function is to reduce acidity and low acidity levels have kicked off your acid reflux in the first place! But sure yeah it's fine to reach for medication to treat today's acid reflux, so long as you realise that to cure acid reflux will take lifestyle changes and some exercises and supplements over a period of months and in some cases years to bring about a cure.

But the good news is that unless you have a major problem with your gastrointestinal tract, such as a burst peptic ulcer or some other major structural damage, then really you can cure yourself of stomach acid reflux, but to do so will take a little time and experimentation.

Finally there is no one way to cure yourself of acid reflux. The best approach is to experiment with different lifestyle changes, exercises and supplements and see what works well for you. The key is to keep an open mind and record your results. Maybe you will try out five or six suggestions from this book and find that only two of them work, well at least that's a start, keep on experimenting and keep your eyes peeled and a stage will come when you are free of acid reflux, but it will only happen when you make a lot of changes to your life and rebalance hour life. Everyone wants to live the same crazy lifestyle and yet be free of acid reflux, but acid reflux is not a disease, it's just a symptoms caused by imbalances in your body!

Also most often when a person suffers from any chronic condition, for a while, some organic damage will be there and some bodily processes will be a little of. For example, the stomach lining or intestinal or oesophageal lining may be damaged organically and it could take several years, yes years, before they're fully healed. Secondly things like enzymes levels might be permanently down and the various gastric processes, of the body, may also be slightly less efficient from usual. Putting this altogether once you have had acid reflux for a while, there will be a tendency for the condition to flare up again, if you're not careful. If your acid reflux has been mild, then you might well be looking at a 100% recovery with no side effects, but in more severe cases stringent lifestyle changes may be required which includes a more strict eye on diet, so as to prevent imbalances form getting out of hand. While it's a pain to have to watch your diet and eat a largely plain and boring diet, it still beats having acid reflux symptoms anyway!

Free Gift

Grab Free Books!!!!!!!!

As a way of saying thank you for downloading this book I would like to give you two free books, which are available exclusively for my readers. The free book "Juicing for Health – 35 Juicing Recipes for Everyday Health Problems", is packed full of useful healthy juice recipes and Success Hacks - 31 Mind-Set Hacks to Increase Productivity and Career Success, is packed full of helpful mind hacks for developing a more dynamic and enjoyable lifestyle!

Please go to http://www.healbodymindandspirit.com/sign-up-page/ and sign up to my subscriber list and you shall receive the free book links via email.

www.ingramcontent.com/pod-product-compliance
Lightning Source LLC
Chambersburg PA
CBHW070120210526
45170CB00013B/825